THE GLOBAL CHALLENGE OF ALZHEIMER'S: THE G-8 DEMENTIA SUMMIT AND BEYOND

HEARING

BEFORE THE

SUBCOMMITTEE ON AFRICA, GLOBAL HEALTH, GLOBAL HUMAN RIGHTS, AND INTERNATIONAL ORGANIZATIONS

OF THE

COMMITTEE ON FOREIGN AFFAIRS
HOUSE OF REPRESENTATIVES

ONE HUNDRED THIRTEENTH CONGRESS

FIRST SESSION

_____

NOVEMBER 21, 2013

_____

Serial No. 113–119

_____

Printed for the use of the Committee on Foreign Affairs

Available via the World Wide Web: http://www.foreignaffairs.house.gov/ or http://www.gpo.gov/fdsys/

_____

U.S. GOVERNMENT PRINTING OFFICE

85–645PDF   WASHINGTON : 2014

For sale by the Superintendent of Documents, U.S. Government Printing Office
Internet: bookstore.gpo.gov   Phone: toll free (866) 512–1800; DC area (202) 512–1800
Fax: (202) 512–2104   Mail: Stop IDCC, Washington, DC 20402–0001

COMMITTEE ON FOREIGN AFFAIRS

EDWARD R. ROYCE, California, *Chairman*

CHRISTOPHER H. SMITH, New Jersey
ILEANA ROS-LEHTINEN, Florida
DANA ROHRABACHER, California
STEVE CHABOT, Ohio
JOE WILSON, South Carolina
MICHAEL T. McCAUL, Texas
TED POE, Texas
MATT SALMON, Arizona
TOM MARINO, Pennsylvania
JEFF DUNCAN, South Carolina
ADAM KINZINGER, Illinois
MO BROOKS, Alabama
TOM COTTON, Arkansas
PAUL COOK, California
GEORGE HOLDING, North Carolina
RANDY K. WEBER SR., Texas
SCOTT PERRY, Pennsylvania
STEVE STOCKMAN, Texas
RON DeSANTIS, Florida
TREY RADEL, Florida
DOUG COLLINS, Georgia
MARK MEADOWS, North Carolina
TED S. YOHO, Florida
LUKE MESSER, Indiana

ELIOT L. ENGEL, New York
ENI F.H. FALEOMAVAEGA, American Samoa
BRAD SHERMAN, California
GREGORY W. MEEKS, New York
ALBIO SIRES, New Jersey
GERALD E. CONNOLLY, Virginia
THEODORE E. DEUTCH, Florida
BRIAN HIGGINS, New York
KAREN BASS, California
WILLIAM KEATING, Massachusetts
DAVID CICILLINE, Rhode Island
ALAN GRAYSON, Florida
JUAN VARGAS, California
BRADLEY S. SCHNEIDER, Illinois
JOSEPH P. KENNEDY III, Massachusetts
AMI BERA, California
ALAN S. LOWENTHAL, California
GRACE MENG, New York
LOIS FRANKEL, Florida
TULSI GABBARD, Hawaii
JOAQUIN CASTRO, Texas

AMY PORTER, *Chief of Staff*   THOMAS SHEEHY, *Staff Director*
JASON STEINBAUM, *Democratic Staff Director*

———————

SUBCOMMITTEE ON AFRICA, GLOBAL HEALTH, GLOBAL HUMAN RIGHTS, AND INTERNATIONAL ORGANIZATIONS

CHRISTOPHER H. SMITH, New Jersey, *Chairman*

TOM MARINO, Pennsylvania
RANDY K. WEBER SR., Texas
STEVE STOCKMAN, Texas
MARK MEADOWS, North Carolina

KAREN BASS, California
DAVID CICILLINE, Rhode Island
AMI BERA, California

CONTENTS

THE GLOBAL CHALLENGE OF ALZHEIMER'S: THE G–8 DEMENTIA SUMMIT AND BEYOND

THURSDAY, NOVEMBER 21, 2013

House of Representatives,
Subcommittee on Africa, Global Health,
Global Human Rights, and International Organizations,
Committee on Foreign Affairs,
Washington, DC.

The subcommittee met, pursuant to notice, at 10:15 a.m., in room 2172 Rayburn House Office Building, Hon. Christopher H. Smith (chairman of the subcommittee) presiding.

Mr. SMITH. We now move to a hearing, pursuant to notice, on the Global Challenge of Alzheimer's: The G–8 Dementia Summit and Beyond. And I recognize myself and then I will go to Dr. Bera.

Good morning. Next month, the United Kingdom will host a meeting of health ministers from G–8 member countries in London to discuss strategies to address the global challenge of Alzheimer's and other forms of dementia. Currently, more than 35 million people worldwide live with some form of dementia. By 2050, this population is projected to triple, in effect, to more than 115 million people. The total cost of dementia, treatment and care is estimated to be somewhere on the order of $604 billion, with about 70 percent of those costs now occurring in Western Europe and North America. As populations age across the globe, today's crisis may become tomorrow's, and will likely become, unless action is taken and cures are found, tomorrow's catastrophe.

Since our subcommittee's June 2011 hearing on this very issue, attention has increasingly turned to dealing with this situation in which people live with dementia, which is more, frankly, than the people living with HIV/AIDS which is about 33 million. Today's hearing is being held in advance of the G–8 Dementia Summit to discuss the policy of the U.S. Government representatives should offer at this conference through recommendations from organizations involved in Alzheimer's and dementia research and treatment.

Many of us have family members, friends, and acquaintances— I don't know anyone who doesn't know someone who suffers from Alzheimer's or some form of dementia. We know the pain of seeing a loved one lose their grip on present circumstances and experience relationships built over decades radically changed forever. Spouses, parents, siblings and other relatives become unable to care for themselves and we are faced with the heartwrenching decision on how best to ensure their care. Sometimes symptoms are too subtle

(1)

to recognize immediately. Sometimes they manifest themselves as sudden changes in personality. However they occur and for whatever reason they occur, these cognitive changes disrupt families and change lives permanently for both the people suffering from these conditions and those who care for them.

The World Health Organization estimates that more than half of global dementia cases are in low and middle income countries where cases are projected to grow. The gross national income per capita in these countries is sometimes less than $1,000. Countries across Africa, Asia, and Latin America are expected to see the rapid growth in dementia cases over the next several decades. In 2010, roughly 53 percent of dementia cases were in low and middle income countries. By 2050, WHO expects 70 percent of all dementia cases to be found in such nations.

In high income countries, family efforts to care for those affected by dementia are supported by the administration of medicines and other professional care services that can be obtained through private insurance or other government-funded programs. In the majority of low and middle income countries, however, low awareness of dementia and its impact are reflected in a lack of comprehensive government policies and public resources aimed at addressing these conditions. As a direct result, care for people living with dementia in these regions is predominately the responsibility of their families.

Support for people with dementia is funded differently across the world. In high income countries, roughly 40 percent of associated costs are borne by the family through informal care, whereas, in low and middle income countries nearly 60 percent of these costs are covered through informal care. Health insurance or other social safety net schemes are typically used in high income countries to alleviate some of the financial burden associated with care for loved ones with dementia. These supports are not widely available or affordable in most low and middle income countries, and the formal social care sectors in these areas are ill equipped. As a result, families in these countries are often required to assume not only the cost of care but also the delivery of that care.

WHO estimates that while 30 percent of people with dementia live in assisted living facilities or nursing homes in high income countries, only 11 percent do so in low and middle income countries. Our Government has worked to enable people in low and middle income countries to enjoy the kind of prosperity those of us in the developed world experience. However, trends indicate that as populations age, they become increasingly prosperous. With immature health systems, however, and inadequate health resources, illnesses that primarily afflict the elderly, such as dementia, risk derailing economic growth as the productive population attempts to care for their older loved ones. Estimates indicate that the proportion of people older than 60 years who will require care will dramatically increase by the year 2050.

We do have an aging planet. The challenge that will face the health ministers gathered in London next month is to find a way to continue to enable increased prosperity in low and middle income countries while taking into account the drain on that prosperity from care for an aging population. Foreign aid to developing countries for health care purposes will change and we need to anticipate that change now before it becomes an overwhelming situation. In the United States and the rest of the developed world, we also must face our own challenges.

As one of our witnesses, Professor Andrea Pfeifer, will testify, the four pillars of the G–8 Dementia Summit are, 1) building public-private cooperation networks; 2) business coordination to prevent dementia; 3) investment in solutions and treatments; and 4) laying the groundwork for the transition to an aging society without dementia. This is indeed a tall order, and cooperation internationally between developed and developing countries, public-private partnerships, and an effective transition to a dementia-free world will be difficult, but not impossible.

We invited experts from the Department of Health and Human Services to attend, who will attend the G–8 summit, to testify at today's hearing, but they have declined, at least for now. We hope to have them appear in a post-Summit hearing to tell us what that gathering achieved and what the U.S. Government role in addressing this global challenge, from their perspective, will be. Meanwhile, we have with us the chief executive officer of one of the world's leading pharmaceutical companies working on Alzheimer's treatment research and two advocates for a more effective response to the challenge of dementia, not only in the United States, but worldwide as well.

The struggle to meet the challenge of HIV/AIDS has been tremendous, and in fact this morning I met with Mark Dybul, the executive director of the Global Fund. The enormous work that is being done through PEPFAR is a great credit to a concerted world effort to mitigate and hopefully eradicate that horrible disease. But we need to, now, in addition to continuing that fight, look at some of these other huge pandemics that we face as global citizens, and certainly dementias, and Alzheimer's is chief among them.

I would like to now yield to Dr. Bera.

Dr. BERA. Thank you Chairman Smith and thank you for—this is an incredibly timely hearing in advance of the G–8 gathering.

I look at Alzheimer's disease from the perspective of being a physician and how it impacts not just the patient but the families and the entire community. And just from personal experience, having cared for both patients as well as family members who are struggling to care for aging parents and so forth, this is an incredibly important issue for us to deal with, particularly when you look at the numbers. I think, if I am not mistaken, over 5 million Americans currently suffer from Alzheimer's disease, and as the baby boomer generation and our population ages it is going to impact America.

The benefit we have though is we have resources and infrastructure to help care and help support those families as they are caring for their loved ones. But as we look at the developing world, as the chairman pointed out, they don't have those resources, so much more of the burden falls onto us as the United States and the developed world to come up with mechanisms and resources to help the developing world.

Within our country, within my home institution of the University of California, Davis, the UC system and our academic research centers, we have to develop an ability to enable the developing countries to better sort through what are treatable causes of dementia versus untreatable causes of dementia. We also have to invest in that research that allows our pharmaceutical companies to come up with the mechanisms and the treatments to, if not cure Alzheimer's at least to help mitigate and slow down the devastating impact of what is right now an irreversible form of dementia.

I was talking to a constituent of mine who is trying to care for her aging parents right now, and again, with the resources we have in the United States she is struggling as her parents get older and older and their dementia gets worse. I can only imagine if you were in a country that didn't have those resources and didn't have those support structures just how difficult it would be.

Again, I applaud the chairman for hosting and holding this hearing. I look forward to hearing what the witnesses have to say. And again I would just encourage all of us here in Congress to think about how we make those investments in research, how we make those investments and enable us to come up with better diagnostic tools and also better therapies and treatment to slow down dementia as well as hopefully one day come up with a cure for Alzheimer's disease. So again, I am looking forward to the testimony.

Mr. SMITH. Thank you very much, Dr. Bera.

Vice Chairman Randy Weber?

Mr. WEBER. Thank you Mr. Chairman. I too appreciate you holding the hearing, and I am going to be very short-winded. Looking forward to the witnesses' testimony. Thank you.

Mr. SMITH. Thank you Mr. Weber.

I would like to now welcome our witnesses, beginning first with, Dr. Andrea Pfeifer is co-founder of AC Immune, in 2003, where she has been CEO since it was founded. She is a member of the WEF Global Agenda Council of Brain and Cognitive Sciences and the CEOi Initiative on Alzheimer's disease. As the former head of Nestle's global research in Switzerland where Professor Pfeifer managed a group of more than 600 people, she brings more than 25 years of senior management experience including broad R&D, business, and international exposure. Dr. Pfeiffer is an international expert in biotechnology and a professor in Switzerland as I mentioned.

Our second witness will be Mr. George Vradenburg who is chairman and co-founder of USAgainstAlzheimer's, an education and advocacy campaign committed to mobilize America to stop Alzheimer's, and convener of the Global CEO Initiative on Alzheimer's. He also helps direct Leaders Engaged on Alzheimer's Disease, a coalition of Alzheimer's serving organization. He has been named by the Secretary of Health and Human Services to serve on the National Alzheimer's Advisory Council to advise on the first of its kind National Alzheimer's Strategic Plan which is mandated from legislation we passed in the last Congress.

Prior to December 2003, Mr. Vradenburg held several senior executive positions in large media companies, and I thank him, because we have met many times that he has been a source of a great deal of input to this subcommittee on what we ought to be doing, and I do greatly appreciate that.

We will then hear from Mr. Matthew Baumgart. He is the senior director of public policy for the Alzheimer's Association. His portfolio includes overseeing state government affairs, the public health project for the Centers for Disease Control, and the public policy department. Prior to joining the Alzheimer's Association, Mr. Baumgart worked for nearly 18 years in the United States Senate. He was legislative director for Senator Barbara Boxer where he supervised the legislative staff, managed all the senator's legislative activities and was her chief legislative strategist. Prior to working for Senator Boxer, Mr. Baumgart worked for over 10 years with then-Senator Joe Biden.

So if we could start with Mr. Vradenburg.

STATEMENT OF MR. GEORGE VRADENBURG, CHAIRMAN AND FOUNDER, USAGAINSTALZHEIMER'S

Mr. VRADENBURG. Thank you very much, Mr. Chairman. Chairman Smith, Mr. Bera and Mr. Weber, I am here today as the convener of the Global CEO Initiative on Alzheimer's. It is a coalition of a number of companies across a number of sectors from pharmaceuticals to medical food to diagnostic companies to financial service companies and home health care companies.

Mr. Chairman, you commented about having met frequently. Much has happened in the last 2½ years since this committee had another hearing on the same subject. We have established a national plan in this country. We have established the rather bold goal of trying to stop this disease by 2025. The World Health Organization has judged Alzheimer's and dementia as a public health priority. OECD has a robust innovation work plan. Professor Peter Piot who headed the U.N. effort on HIV/AIDS has called now for a global plan against Alzheimer's and dementia, viewing it as a challenge to the 21st century much like HIV/AIDS was at the end of the 20th century. And as you mentioned, next month at the invitation of Prime Minister David Cameron, representatives from G–8 nations are gathering in London for the first ever G–8 Global Dementia Summit.

More than a dozen years ago, the G–8 met in Okinawa to commit to a global effort to fight HIV/AIDS. It was a turning point in the world's attention to that disease. And the United States during the course of the Bush administration stepped up the Global Fund and the PEPFAR, as you mentioned, and it was proven to be extraordinarily successful even as we still have more to do. A similar G–8 commitment to address Alzheimer's and dementia would make this a pivotal moment in the history of this disease as historians write of the battle against this disease in the 21st century.

I have urged the U.S. delegation to use the G–8 summit to press for the development of a global plan to stop Alzheimer's, and I am urging today that the U.S. delegation begin to lay the foundation for a global fund to finance that effort by calling on nations to contribute 1 percent of their national costs of caring for those with the disease to a global fund to stop it. So for the United States, if costs are roughly $200 billion a year, a 1-percent contribution would represent $2 billion a year.

A global plan must be actionable, goal oriented, and updated regularly. It has got to be designed, it seems to me, to reinforce national plans and strategies. It has got to be appropriately financed. And it has to enjoy the strong and sustained backing of government leaders, not just from the G–8 nations, but from the entire range of low, middle income, and high income countries because the footprint of this disease is, as you have emphasized, Mr. Chairman, much broader than the eight nations that are going to be represented in London. So London should be regarded with the G–8 as a first step.

It seems to me that a plan should focus on critical and emerging areas in need of global coordination, new financing to finance Alzheimer's research, drug development and care, for example, through a global fund, but not limited to a global fund. Multi-national high-performance infrastructures for Alzheimer's longitudinal studies and clinical trials to identify the means of both pharmacological and nonpharmacological interventions to prevent this disease are other key elements.

A third element of this plan has to address the critical issues of basic and regulatory science such as the scientific development and regulatory qualification of predictive AD biomarkers. The fourth element of this plan, it seems to me, has to deal with the new age of technology, and we need to develop globally interoperative, technology-driven techniques to thoroughly and expeditiously exploit the voluminous amounts of big data that are being generated by genomic science and electronic health records. This needs to be turned to discovering the mechanisms of action of this disease, those at risk for the disease and cures for those diseased. And of course it has to deal with care innovations.

As you mentioned, Mr. Chairman, every country has dealt with care of those with Alzheimer's in quite different ways. New technology-assisted mechanisms of monitoring care management, of care coordination, and potentially care quality controls, seem to me to permit us now to exchange information with the rest of the world in terms of the innovations that are needed to assure quality care across care settings in stages of the disease, and to make sure they are efficiently delivered. If we commit to these efforts, the potential value to the public is huge.

A recent report by RTI International found that if we make certain reforms in our infrastructure, we can reduce the cost and risk of developing Alzheimer's therapy by over half, speed up by nearly 18 months the time to get a therapy to patients, reduce by millions the number of dementia years of Alzheimer's, and save hundreds of billions of dollars in public cost. This is just in the United States.

Excuse me, I am getting over a cold as you can hear, and so I apologize if my voice breaks like a 14-year-old boy.

These findings underscore what is possible when the appropriate level of resources, focus, and planning are directed at this problem. As JFK, whose assassination we recognize tomorrow, emphasized when he made his moonshot speech, we do not set goals and regard them as easy. We set goals that are hard and we do that because it will mobilize our resources, our intellect, and our focus to solve the problem in front of us. That is what we need now. Thus, I am urging the U.S. and other nations to develop a global action plan along these lines starting at the G–8 summit.

The global CEO Initiative on Alzheimer's will be convening a meeting on December 12 in London following the December 11 global Summit with the representatives of the key G–8 nations, as well as with industry and scientific leaders, in order to turn the political commitments that are made at the G–8 summit into action plans in 2014.

I am also urging the U.S. to be not only more actively participatory in these international efforts, but to lead these international efforts. As you pointed out, Mr. Chairman, the United States ended up leading the effort against the HIV/AIDS. We didn't just participate and allow others to lead. We took the leadership against the global pandemic, and in fact much of the progress that has been made has clearly been a global effort, but much of the progress has been made because of the leadership of the United States.

So the United States can lead not just at the G–8 summit. There are some workshops that are contemplated in 2014 to follow up on the G–8 summit, but there is also continuing work at the OECD in which the United States has not been an active and engaged participant. And we need to ensure that while the Prime Minister of England is the President of the G–8s for this year, his presidency ends at the end of the year and we need leadership that will continue this effort at a global level after December 31. And so the United States is, of course, the natural leader in these areas and should take the lead as we move forward after the end of this year.

And I would encourage you, Mr. Chairman. You have been active and you have focused on this important issue, but international parliamentarians are eager to establish a regular, ongoing dialogue and conversation among parliamentarians about what ought to be done. Both in Europe and Japan, we have talked to them. They are ready, willing and able to establish with you, Mr. Chairman, an international parliamentarian group that will begin to focus on this disease and not allow it to rest simply with the executive branches of the various countries.

And finally, on research funding, I would urge all of you to support increases in our own NIH budget, generally, as well as for Alzheimer's research. Senators Collins and Klobuchar, last night, introduced a resolution in the Senate to double Alzheimer's research from its current roughly $500 million to $1 billion in Fiscal 2015, and then over a period of years to increase that level of investment to $2 billion.

I would urge a similar action in the House, and with your leadership, Mr. Chairman, I think that would be a formidable effort. It is a bipartisan effort. This is a disease that killed Ronald Reagan. It killed Sargent Shriver. This disease knows no party. The costs of this disease to our fiscal and our entitlement programs knows no party, and this is an area where I think the United States, as it has done in the past with HIV/AIDS, can do it again with Alzheimer's and dementia. So I thank you very much for the opportunity to be here this morning, and I thank you again, Mr. Chairman, for your leadership in this space.

[The prepared statement of Mr. Vradenburg follows:]

Testimony of George Vradenburg
Chairman, USAgainstAlzheimer's
Convener, The Global CEO Initiative on Alzheimer's Disease

Before the House Subcommittee on Africa, Global Health,
Global Human Rights and International Organizations

The Global Challenge of Alzheimer's: The G-8 Dementia Summit and Beyond

Thursday, November 21, 2013

Chairman Smith, Ranking Member Bass and other members of the Committee – Thank you very much for calling this important and well-timed hearing, just a few weeks before the landmark G8 Global Dementia Summit called for by British Prime Minister Cameron.

A little more than two years ago, this committee held a similar hearing exploring the global impact of Alzheimer's disease. At that time, the United States Congress had recently passed the National Alzheimer's Project Act, and the Administration was working to implement the law. Much has changed since then, and this activity is not limited to the United States.

In addition to the launch of the U.S. National Plan, which sets as its first goal the prevention and effective treatment of Alzheimer's by 2025, nearly a dozen other nations have adopted national strategies of their own, as have a number of regions, provinces, and states. The World Health Organization (WHO) last year declared dementia a "public health priority," noting that the nearly 36 million people estimated to be living with this disease in 2010 would double by 2030 and more than triple by 2050 if the current trajectory remains unchanged[1].

Thankfully, the future remains unwritten, and we have seen time and again that when the world unites to tackle a grave threat to our health and well-being, the unthinkable becomes the possible. In 2000, at the G8 Summit in Okinawa, world leaders recognized the grave threat posed by HIV/AIDS and resolved to do something about it. Today, through programs like the Global Fund to Treat AIDS, Tuberculosis and Malaria and the President's Emergency Plan for AIDS Relief (PEPFAR), millions of people worldwide are being treated, and future cases are being prevented. In watershed remarks delivered in March 2012, Professor Peter Piot, who led the United Nation's AIDS effort, called dementia one of the largest neglected global health issues of this generation and called for a global effort similar to that waged against HIV/AIDS.[2]

The Global Action Plan

Today, I am here to reinforce Professor Piot's call for a global action plan and to urge this subcommittee and this House to be a champion and driver behind this action. I also urge that as part of this effort, we lay a foundation to establish a patient-centered Global Fund to Stop Alzheimer's, focused on delivering the resources necessary to develop and deliver therapies and treatments and to support patients and caregivers in this struggle. The time is now to capitalize on this unprecedented level of international momentum and resolve to stopping

---

[1] See: http://www.who.int/mental_health/publications/dementia_report_2012/en/
[2] See: http://www.alzheimers.org.uk/site/scripts/news_article.php?newsID=1169

Alzheimer's disease and dementia and to commit the nations of the world to a Global Action Plan to stop Alzheimer's disease. In order to be as effective as were the efforts against HIV/AIDS, such a Plan must:

- Be **comprehensive, goal oriented,** and **informed by experts** in science, drug development and discovery, care delivery, financing, technology, insurance and other areas; and be **regularly updated** so as to assure a sustained unity of purpose as well as accountability for progress against goals;

- **Reinforce plans** developed or being developed by individual nations or regions;

- Be **financed with the appropriate amount of resources** necessary to achieve its goals and objectives; and

- Enjoy the **strong and sustained backing of government leaders at the highest levels, acting through national, multilateral and global bodies.**

Elements of the Plan

Absent these principles, it is highly unlikely that any global action plan could be effective. Earlier this month, the Global CEO Initiative on Alzheimer's Disease, the New York Academy of Sciences, and the National Institute on Aging convened the *Alzheimer's Disease Summit: the*

Path to 2025. This two-day conference brought together leading researchers, drug developers, investors, technology experts, policy makers and others to help flesh out a clearer path as to research priorities and other innovations necessary to stop Alzheimer's disease by 2025. During this meeting, three topics in particular emerged as priorities:

- New mechanisms to finance Alzheimer's research and drug discovery efforts;

- Use of a standing global clinical trial system to reduce the time, cost, and risk associated with clinical trials; and

- Better use of information technology to more fully utilize the "big data" now emerging in electronic health records and the human genome that may hold a key to our success.

Not a single one of these actions can be the exclusive domain of any one single country. On the contrary, absent a truly global commitment and high degree of international collaboration, it is difficult to envision success in any of these areas. For example:

- The absence of interoperability has hampered the ability to connect the databases of the World-Wide Alzheimer's Disease Neuroimaging Initiative (ADNI).

- Enrollment in global Alzheimer's disease clinical trials – already a labor-intensive process, particularly as researchers look to conduct trials in patients with only mild symptoms or who are presymptomatic – is made even more lengthy and costly absent a standing global Alzheimer's clinical trials network.

- Research and development – from the basic levels to late stage translational and clinical science – can be duplicative absent high levels of coordination and collaboration, wasting scarce resource dollars, both public and private, in the process.

The Benefits of Greater Investment & Coordination

Despite these challenges, a recent study by RTI International released during the *Alzheimer's Disease Summit* makes clear the immense benefits possible through accelerating Alzheimer's research and development. Specifically, the report recommends an increased focus on several key areas – including a streamlined process to enroll in clinical trials, a stronger and more versatile clinical trials system able to test and qualify Alzheimer's disease biomarkers, and higher levels of collaboration to reduce the time, cost, and risk of therapy development – to accelerate the development of Alzheimer's therapies.

Were such infrastructure changes to be adopted, the analysis shows they could significantly reduce the overall cost of Alzheimer's drug development from about $5.7 *billion* under the current environment to the still high yet far more manageable $2 *billion.* In addition, such reforms would shave nearly a year-and-a-half off of current drug development timeline, largely by allowing potential therapies to "fail faster" during less-costly earlier stages of research, thereby maximizing the likelihood that compounds entering late-stage trials are likely to succeed.

This significant reduction in time and cost is impressive, but the benefits don't end here. If we are successful in accelerating the pace of discovery and delivering disease-modifying drugs to patients earlier, this would likely result in an estimated 7 million fewer cases of dementia in the United States alone during the 15 year timeframe from 2025 to 2040.

Potential Reduction in the Number of Cases of Dementia in the United States with an Improved Technical and Research Infrastructure

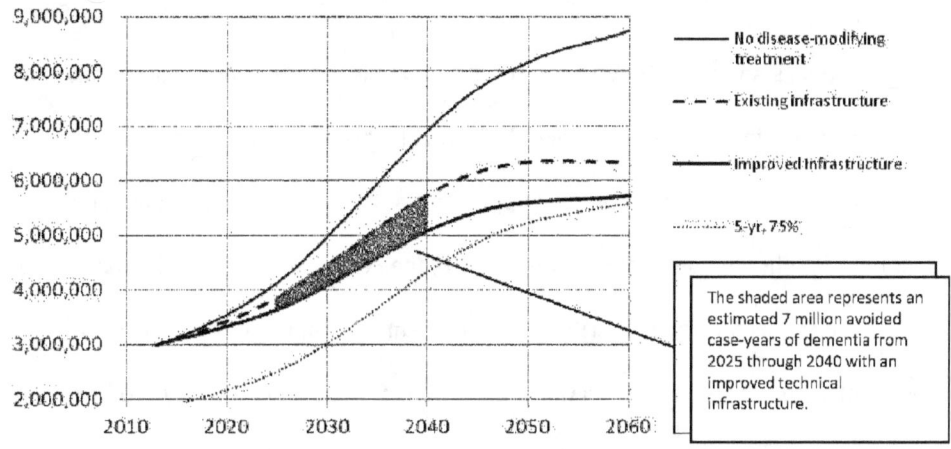

The shaded area represents an estimated 7 million avoided case-years of dementia from 2025 through 2040 with an improved technical infrastructure.

The Call to Action

The outputs of the recent 'The Path to 2025' summit and the RTI report provide the foundation upon which the G8, the G20, the OECD, the WHO, and other stakeholders can build upon to develop the Global Action Plan to Stop Alzheimer's disease and, ultimately, a catalytic global

fund. The G8 Summit and the planned follow-on workshops to occur throughout 2014 provide

the process through which such a plan can be crafted, refined, and finalized. I urge the United

States delegation to the Summit to lead this push and to commit to a set of time-bound

milestones to develop the plan in the coming year. I also urge the U.S. government to fully

engage in all related international pursuits, particularly those by the G8, the G20, the

Organization for Economic Cooperation and Development (OECD) and the WHO, that are

focused on Alzheimer's and dementia. Specifically, I call upon our government to more fully

participate in the work being done by the OECD in this important area.

From a Congressional standpoint, I encourage this subcommittee to continue doing what you

are doing in conducting invaluable oversight of U.S. and global efforts to address the

Alzheimer's crisis. I also urge you to consider opportunities to work with a growing body of

parliamentarians in other nations – particularly the UK, the European Union, and Japan – who

are also deeply interested in stopping Alzheimer's and dementia and willing to engage in

dialogue with fellow parliamentarians on this topic. Such efforts could be highly productive in

spurring and sustaining the commitment of governments to the Global Action Plan.

Finally, I will close with one thought on research financing, recognizing the continued fiscal

challenges our nation and others are facing. I've said many times that we don't have a choice

as to whether or not we will pay for the costs of Alzheimer's and dementia. Taxpayers are

paying dearly today, to the tune of about $140 billion in annual entitlement costs of care shouldered by Medicare and Medicaid, a price tag that will skyrocket over the coming years. On the flip side, even despite some recent modest yet important infusions of funding for Alzheimer's disease research, our public commitment to this goal languishes at about $500 million annually, about 0.36 percent of the amount spent every year on care.

If global governments would commit 1 percent of their annual costs of caring for Alzheimer's patients, this would begin moving toward a level of Alzheimer's disease research funding commensurate with the scope of the challenge. A portion of this funding could also be used to seed a Global Fund to Stop Alzheimer's disease and to implement a Global Action Plan to Stop Alzheimer's disease, similar to efforts waged against HIV/AIDS. Here at home, a growing number of lawmakers and advocates have been promoting a near-term doubling of the Alzheimer's and dementia budget at the NIH, a move that would make significant progress in this direction. I urge the members of this committee to strongly consider this idea.

Thank you, again, for conducting this hearing. Despite the challenges that lay ahead, I remain optimistic that our nation and our world can stop Alzheimer's disease if we commit ourselves to this ambitious goal, and I urge you to advance a Global Action Plan to Stop Alzheimer's to drive this work.

———————

Mr. SMITH. Mr. Vradenburg, thank you very much for your leadership and for your extraordinarily crisp and incisive testimony with very concrete recommendations. And you are right. We just have to lead. I think your point was very well taken.

Mr. VRADENBURG. The scarcest commodity in this field, Chairman, is leadership.

Mr. SMITH. Thank you.

Mr. Baumgart?

STATEMENT OF MR. MATTHEW BAUMGART, SENIOR DIRECTOR OF PUBLIC POLICY, ALZHEIMER'S ASSOCIATION

Mr. BAUMGART. Thank you very much, Mr. Chairman. I would ask that my written testimony be included in the record.

Mr. SMITH. Without objection, so ordered.

Mr. BAUMGART. I want to thank you and the members of this committee for holding this important hearing today on the global dementia crisis and the upcoming G–8 summit on dementia research. Mr. Chairman, the Alzheimer's Association is the world's largest private, nonprofit funder of Alzheimer's research, and we are also the world's leading organization on Alzheimer's care and support. Every day, we see what this devastating disease does to families. We see what it does to individuals. And we see the heavy toll it takes on family members.

I want to tell you one particular story of somebody that we have worked with and we have helped. His name is Randy and he lives in California, is the caregiver for his mother who has Alzheimer's disease. And in Randy's words, I know there is going to be a problem when Mom goes into the bathroom and doesn't come out for a long time, because she is either too embarrassed or too proud to ask for help. Randy continues by saying, I know then that I am going to have to clean up not only Mom but the entire bathroom. And Randy says he finds himself often asking, who would have believed that I would be changing the diapers of the woman who changed mine?

That is Alzheimer's disease. It is not just a little memory loss. It is not a normal part of aging. It is a devastating disease that means the loss of anything and everything you have ever known. And as you noted, there are now over 35 million people worldwide living with dementia, over 5 million here in the United States, as Mr. Bera noted. Those numbers could triple by mid-century; 115 million people globally could be living with dementia.

In addition to the toll that Alzheimer's disease takes on families, it also takes a toll on government budgets. A study published in the New England Journal of Medicine earlier this year found that dementia was the most costly disease in America, costing more than cancer and heart disease. And the estimates are that 70 percent of the costs of caring for people with the disease are borne by taxpayers through the Medicare and Medicaid programs. Globally, as you noted, in 2010 the cost of dementia was $604 billion. If dementia were a country, it would be the 18th largest global economy.

Mr. Chairman, a global crisis requires a global response. And here in the United States we began that response in 2010 when Congress unanimously passed, through your leadership, the National Alzheimer's Project Act, which requires the Federal Government for the first time ever to have a national strategy on how to address this crisis. This leadership, here in the United States must now be extended to a global effort, starting with the G–8 summit in London on December 11th.

The G–8 summit provides a unique opportunity to tackle dementia on a global scale. If it is to be successful, we at the Alzheimer's Association believe that the G–8 nations must develop a shared vision for addressing and driving dementia research over the next decade. Specifically, that means there must be a commitment from each country of the G–8 to increase its own level of dementia research funding commensurate with the level of the crisis. It means identifying additional innovative research opportunities and mechanisms such as public-private partnerships. It means improved coordination in dementia research across governments, the research community, nonprofit organizations as well as private industry. And it means a commitment to create an environment in each country that will train, attract and develop the very best scientists.

Finally, we believe that each G–8 nation must commit to developing its own national dementia plan much as the United States, the United Kingdom, and France, among the G–8 nations, have already done. But let us be clear. The G–8 summit is not the end of the process, it is only the beginning of the process. As important as it is for the G–8 nations to develop a shared vision, a shared commitment and a shared strategy, it is equally important that they commit to action following the summit. A vision, a commitment and a strategy must be implemented if we are going to succeed globally.

In closing, Mr. Chairman, I would like to go back to something that you mentioned, and that is, past efforts on global cooperation. Because of medical research and medical innovation globally and cooperatively, millions of people around the globe have better lives. It has improved the lives of people who are living with heart disease, with HIV/AIDS, and with cancer. Now is the time to make dementia a global priority, and the G–8 summit provides a historic opportunity to do so. Thank you.

[The prepared statement of Mr. Baumgart follows:]

www.alz.org

Public Policy Office
1212 New York Avenue, NW
Suite 800
Washington, DC 20005-6105

202 393 7737 **p**
866 865 0270 **f**

alzheimer's ♋ association

Testimony of Matthew Baumgart, Senior Director of Public Policy of the Alzheimer's Association
The Global Challenge of Alzheimer's: The G-8 Dementia Summit and Beyond

Subcommittee on Africa, Global Health, Global Human Right, and International Organizations
Committee on Foreign Affairs
United States House of Representatives

November 21, 2013

Good morning Chairman Smith, Ranking Member Bass, and members of the Subcommittee. Thank you for the opportunity to testify on the global challenge of Alzheimer's disease and the opportunity for global progress with the upcoming G8 Summit on dementia research.

Founded in 1980, the Alzheimer's Association is the world's leading voluntary health organization in Alzheimer's care, support, and research. Our mission is to eliminate Alzheimer's disease and other dementias through the advancement of research; to provide and enhance care and support for all affected; and to reduce the risk of dementia through the promotion of brain health. As the world's largest nonprofit funder of Alzheimer's research, the Association is committed to accelerating progress of new treatments, preventions, and ultimately a cure. Through our funded projects and partnerships, we have been a part of every major research advancement over the past 30 years. And, through our work to enhance care and provide support for all those affected by Alzheimer's, we have helped millions of individuals living with the disease and their families.

The Global Impact of Alzheimer's

Alzheimer's disease is a global public health crisis. This crisis is placing – and will increasingly place – an enormous strain on families, the health care system, and government budgets of nations around the world. Current estimates indicate that about 36 million people worldwide are living with dementia, and when we reach the middle of the 21st century, there will be 115 million people living with dementia. Dementia has been creating an enormous burden in North America and Western Europe. Increasingly, that burden is spreading to low- and moderate-income countries. Between 2010 and 2050, the number of people with dementia in low- and moderate-income countries is expected to quadruple – and the proportion of worldwide dementia cases in low- and moderate-income countries will increase from 58 percent to over 70 percent.

the compassion to care, the leadership to conquer

In its 2010 annual report – *The Global Economic Impact of Dementia* – Alzheimer's Disease International (ADI) reported that the global cost of dementia totaled $604 billion in 2010, amounting to one percent of global Gross Domestic Product (GDP). If dementia were a country, it would be the 18th largest global economy.

Research shows that most people currently living with dementia have not received a formal diagnosis. In the United States, as many as half of the over 5 million individuals with Alzheimer's have not been diagnosed. And, in India, a study found that nearly 90 percent of those with dementia remain unidentified. In total, ADI concluded in 2011 that as many as 28 million of the 36 million people living with dementia throughout the world have not been diagnosed and therefore do not have access to the treatment, care, and organized support that a formal diagnosis enables.

The global burden of this devastating disease was further underscored in this year's ADI report on long-term care. The report found that as the world's population ages, the traditional system of informal care by family, friends, and community will require much greater support. Today, it is estimated that 13 percent of people aged 60 or over require long-term care. Between 2010 and 2050, the total number of older people with care needs will nearly triple from 101 million to 277 million. And people with dementia are a large portion of that number. In the United States, for example, nearly 65 percent of nursing home residents have dementia.

Global Research Efforts

The global Alzheimer's crisis requires a global response. And while the Alzheimer's Association is a U.S.-based organization, we are committed to working globally to eliminate Alzheimer's disease. No single organization can surmount a challenge as great as Alzheimer's. To help achieve our vision of a world without Alzheimer's, the Association partners with key government, industry, and academic stakeholders around the world. We believe in the value of collaboration and that it can be the catalyst toward achieving disease-modifying treatments, prevention, and ultimately a cure.

The Association formula for progress rests on four pillars: funding, collaborating with investigators, sharing data, and overcoming barriers to progress. The first pillar is the Alzheimer's Association International Grant Program. Typically 10 to 15 percent of our grant funds are spent outside the United States. Currently, we fund active grants in 21 countries, and have funded research in 28 countries overall.

The second pillar of the Alzheimer's Association program is encouraging increased cooperation between scientists. The Association convenes the largest meeting of Alzheimer's scientists every year – the Alzheimer's Association International Conference

(AAIC). This year in Boston, over 5,000 scientists attended AAIC to share research results, compare progress, and develop new working collaborations to advance the fight against the disease.

The third pillar of our program is the sharing of information. We initiated the International Society to Advance Alzheimer's Research and Treatment (ISTAART), a professional society that encourages networking among Alzheimer's researchers so they can share their findings and learn from each other. We also publish *Alzheimer's & Dementia*, which has been rated as the highest impact dementia journal and the third in impact among 191 clinical neurology journals. *Alzheimer's & Dementia* provides a single peer-reviewed publication for the global scientific community to report the latest research developments and results.

The fourth and final pillar of our global research efforts is investing in large-scale projects to overcome common barriers in the field of Alzheimer's. Projects include TrialMatch™ -- an individualized clinical trial matching service for people with Alzheimer's and other dementias -- World Wide Alzheimer's Disease Neuroimaging Initiative (WW-ADNI) -- the umbrella organization of neuroimaging initiatives being conducted around the world -- and the Cerebrospinal Fluid (CSF) Quality Control Program -- which brings together laboratories across the globe with the aim of standardizing the measurement of potential Alzheimer's biomarkers.

Changing the Trajectory of Alzheimer's

As I mentioned, no single organization can surmount a challenge as great as Alzheimer's. And no matter how important and critical the Association's global efforts are, we will not be successful without a serious and sustained commitment from the federal government. In 2010, the bipartisan National Alzheimer's Project Act (NAPA) (P.L. 111-375) passed Congress unanimously, requiring the creation of an annually-updated strategic National Alzheimer's Plan to help those with the disease and their families today and to change the trajectory of the disease for the future. The Plan is required to include an evaluation of all federally-funded efforts in Alzheimer's research, care, and services -- along with their outcomes. NAPA will allow Congress to assess whether the nation is meeting the challenges of this disease for families, communities, and the economy. Through its annual review process, NAPA will, for the first time, enable Congress and the American people to answer this simple question: are we making satisfactory progress in the fight against Alzheimer's?

As mandated by NAPA, the Secretary of Health and Human Services, in collaboration with the Advisory Council on Alzheimer's Research, Care, and Services, developed the first-ever *National Plan to Address Alzheimer's Disease* in May 2012, with an update released in June 2013. The Advisory Council, composed of both federal members and expert non-federal members, is an integral part of the planning process as it advises the Secretary in developing and evaluating the annual Plan, makes recommendations to the Secretary and Congress, and assists in coordinating the work of federal agencies involved in Alzheimer's research, care, and services.

Having a Plan with measurable outcomes is important. But unless there are resources to implement the Plan and the will to follow through on its action steps, we cannot hope to make much progress. If we are going to succeed in the fight against Alzheimer's, Congress must provide the resources the scientists need. A disease-modifying or preventive therapy would not only save millions of lives but would save billions of dollars in health care costs. According to an economic model developed by the non-partisan health econometrics firm, The Lewin Group, a treatment that delayed the onset of Alzheimer's by five years (a treatment similar to anti-cholesterol drugs) would reduce Medicare and Medicaid spending on people with Alzheimer's nearly in half in 2050.

Because of the Plan, the National Institutes of Health (NIH) finally has created a blueprint for Alzheimer's research that includes a timeline and milestones toward the goal of preventing and effectively treating Alzheimer's by 2025. And, we are grateful for the additional resources that NIH has provided for Alzheimer's research in the past couple of years, including the recent announcement by NIH Director Francis Collins that $45 million in additional funding would go to Alzheimer's research. These are, however, baby steps. According to a study published earlier this year in the *New England Journal of Medicine,* dementia is the most expensive disease in America. We do not have a commitment on research funding commensurate with this crisis. For every $27,000 that Medicare and Medicaid spend caring for individuals with Alzheimer's, NIH spends only $100 on Alzheimer's research. Scientists fundamentally believe that we have the ideas, the technology, and the will to develop new Alzheimer's interventions. But progress depends on a prioritized scientific agenda backed up by the necessary resources to carry it out.

The scientists have determined that additional research on Alzheimer's is a priority, and they have asked Congress to provide an additional $80 million in funding for fiscal year 2014. Their budget request reflects the urgent need for Alzheimer's research and the scientific opportunity that now exists. It is vital that Congress support the research projects the scientists at NIH deem necessary.

What Needs to Be Done at the G8 Meeting

But just as the Alzheimer's Association cannot go it alone, so, too, the United States cannot go it alone. Congress recognized this when it passed NAPA, which requires the Secretary of Health and Human Services to coordinate with international bodies "to integrate and inform the fight against Alzheimer's globally." In 2012, the World Health Organization called dementia a public health priority, and now dementia research must become a global priority. The G8 Summit in London on December 11 is a unique opportunity for international leaders to tackle dementia on a global scale, and it presents a historic opportunity to transform our commitment and approach.

The Alzheimer's Association believes that if the G8 is going to make a difference in dementia policy and research, then the G8 nations must develop a collaborative, global action plan for government, industry, and nonprofit organizations to work collaboratively and effectively on an international scale, with appropriate infrastructure and policies in place that break down barriers to effective research.

Specifically, it is vital that the G8 nations develop a shared vision for driving dementia research over the next decade to ensure the development of effective treatments for people worldwide. This vision should include a commitment by each country to increase its own funding into the cause, cure, and prevention of dementia to a level proportionate to the human and economic burden of the disease. It must include identifying additional, innovative funding models, such as public-private partnerships. It must involve improved coordination in research efforts among governments, the research community, non-profit organizations, and industry. And, it must include a commitment to creating a research environment that attracts, develops, and trains the very best scientists, clinicians, and health care professionals.

Finally, each G8 country must commit to having a national Alzheimer's and dementia plan of its own, just as the United States, the United Kingdom, and France have – plans that evaluate progress and share results to determine the best practices and most effective policies.

Moving Beyond the G8 Summit

But, let's be clear: the G8 summit is not the end of the process; it is only the beginning. As important as it is for the G8 countries to develop a shared vision, a shared commitment, and a shared strategy for moving forward, it is equally important that there be concerted and sustained action following the Summit. The vision, the commitment, and the strategy must be implemented if we are to succeed.

The G8 Summit must also be just the start of a wider global conversation about making dementia a global priority. Other global bodies, including the World Health Organization through efforts such as the Global Action Plan on the Prevention and Control of Noncommunicable Diseases, must work to support not only increased dementia research but also the development of care and support systems in low- and moderate-income countries to relieve the dramatically growing impact of dementia on their health and social systems.

Mr. Chairman, medical research has transformed the lives of millions living with heart disease, stroke, HIV/AIDS, and cancer. Now is the time to make dementia a priority.

Thank you again for inviting me to participate in this important discussion about the global impact of Alzheimer's disease and the G8 Summit on dementia research. The Alzheimer's Association commends the Subcommittee for holding today's hearing, and we look forward to continuing to work with you to do all we can to improve the lives of those living with Alzheimer's as well as of those who care for them.

————————

Mr. SMITH. Thank you very much for your leadership and your testimony as well, and it couldn't have been better stated. I do hope that the administration, and I think it is, is paying close attention to what the advocates who really walk point on this issue, and you two are chief among them. We did invite HHS to be here. I am a little bit chagrined that they are not here, but I give them the benefit of the doubt, as long as they do the right thing. And we will be doing a follow-up hearing on what we do next after whatever the G–8 comes to conclusions about in terms of what their plan of action will be.

And I think your point, the parallels with the HIV/AIDS pandemic, is just so compelling. I remember when Henry Hyde sat here and he was the prime sponsor of the Bush-backed bill, he brought in conservatives, moderates, liberals across the board. The same thing happened over on the Senate side. But PEPFAR looked like Mount Everest when it was first introduced, and now looking back it was like, well, why wasn't that an easy pass? It wasn't, but it took leadership. And our hope, and you both have said it, how important it is that we lead. That the G–8 summit is only a beginning, it is not the end. It is not a little check in the box and then you move on to something else. This has to be serious and sustained.

And we do have Dr. Pfeifer on line ready to testify, and so if we could go to her, and then we will go to questions.

STATEMENT OF ANDREA PFEIFER, PH.D., CHIEF EXECUTIVE OFFICER, AC IMMUNE (APPEARING VIA VIDEOCONFERENCE)

Ms. PFEIFER. Mr. Chairman Smith, members of the committee, I am honored to be invited today to address the members of the Committee on Foreign Affairs as you consider potential policies for discussion at the upcoming G–8 Dementia Summit in London. Perhaps I will make a few opening remarks. For the past 10 years I have built from scratch the company AC Immune, which is focused on developing potentials, therapies and diagnostics for Alzheimer's. We have some notable success of a drug, Crenezumab, invented by us and developed by Genentech, which was selected to be tested in the world's first ever prevention trial for Alzheimer's funded under President Obama's NAPA initiative.

My passion as a scientist to find a therapy for this terrible disease is matched by my determination to engage with key policymakers such as yourselves to pull together all the key elements of a global action plan similar to what the world established 30 years ago when faced with the HIV/AIDS epidemic. In my view, the challenges of Alzheimer's today are on the same scale if not greater.

Previous speakers have commented on the hard, basic facts on Alzheimer's disease in the U.S. I would like to draw your attention to the European situation. We do face exactly the same problem with Alzheimer's in Europe as in the U.S. The disease is a terrible human burden with a massive economic impact. However, at the same time it is heavily under-researched and the research is under-financed. An estimated 8.5 million Europeans currently suffer from the disease. As in other countries, the number is projected to nearly double every 20 years as a result of an aging population. Only very few countries as, for example, France, Sweden, and the

UK have established policies and strategic plans similar to a NAPA in the U.S.

We are a drug-developing company with a dream on the goal to find an ultimate cure for Alzheimer's disease facing several major challenges. We do not know the exact cause of the disease and the molecular basis. We know, however, that there are proteins in the body, namely, beta-amyloid and tau which are ultimately involved in the disease. One of the stumbling blocks of Alzheimer's treatments seem to be the time of clinical intervention. Learning from the recent failures of drugs in clinical development, the scientific community and industry strives toward very early pre-symptomatic intervention and even prevention of the disease.

Unfortunately, as you can imagine, delivering a therapy to people before they are even showing symptoms implicates huge clinical trials with large patient numbers, incredibly long timelines and costs that exceed the infrastructure and possibilities of a single company even if it is a big pharma company. Some of the most serious challenges which we only are able to tackle with common efforts are the need for early diagnostic and well-accepted biomarkers to accelerate clinical trials, access to patients and the need to share data, regulatory hurdles and funding.

Europe has very important activities ongoing and I will mention three important ones. First, the European Medicines Agency released a concept paper on the need to revise the guidelines on medicines for treatment of Alzheimer's, for public consultation until January. A second initiative is a private-public partnership for AD clinical trials, EPOCH AD, focusing on cooperation between government, industry and academia to enhance the drug development process. Third, the European Commission also created the European Innovation Partnership, EIP, on Active and Healthy Aging, a stakeholder-driven approach to innovation in its domain. All of these activities are highly welcome and can serve as a wonderful platform on which a global Alzheimer's action plan can be built on.

I applause for UK Prime Minister Cameron for conveying the first G–8 summit on Dementia to work on the four already-mentioned pillars. Building cooperation networks among governments, regulators, the private sector and nonprofits; sharing of knowledge leading to prevention of dementia; investment in solution and treatments; and laying the foundation for transition to an aging society without dementia.

I am particular enthusiastic and optimistic about the potential for greater levels of public-private partnership not limited to one nation or region but rather spanning the world. Such efforts are necessary if we are to achieve our shared goal of defeating Alzheimer's disease and dementia which affects the entire globe and just national borders. It is a global crisis that merits a global response.

In conclusion, it is my earnest desire to convey to the committee, Mr. Chairman, that we need the inspiring leadership of the United States Government to play a key role and be a role model in facing one of the most severe and complex challenge of the 21st century. The U.S. could play a cohesive role in helping to join hands through the G–8 summit and extending the message across the

OECD. The CEO Initiative on Alzheimer's Disease spearheaded by George Vradenburg can be the key catalyst of all of these efforts.

Although many differences exist within the international community, we share an important goal: Finding a cure for Alzheimer's disease and eliminating the personal, financial and social burden of this disease. I remain confident that with the united forces and the lead of your nation in a global action plan we can achieve this goal. Thank you again, Mr. Chairman, for this hearing, and I welcome questions.

[The prepared statement of Ms. Pfeifer follows:]

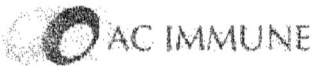

Testimony of Prof. Andrea Pfeifer
Chief Executive Officer
AC IMMUNE

HOUSE COMMITTEE ON FOREIGN AFFAIRS
Subcommittee on Africa, Global Health, Global Human Rights, and International
Organizations
259A Ford House Office Building
Washington, D.C. 20515

The Global Challenge of Alzheimer's: The G-8 Dementia Summit and Beyond
November 21, 2013

Good morning ladies and gentlemen.

Thank you Chairman Smith, Ranking Member Bass and other members of the Committee. I am Dr. Andrea Pfeifer, the CEO of AC Immune, a biopharmaceutical company based in Switzerland developing drugs against Alzheimer's disease. Founded in 2003, AC Immune takes pride in the discovery of Crenezumab, which is being developed by Genentech with support from NIH for the first ever preventive clinical trial in Colombia and the US. AC Immune has three clinical trial programs, four preclinical and a diagnostic program. I am honored to be invited today to address the members of the Committee on Foreign Affairs as you consider potential policies for discussion at the upcoming G8 Dementia Summit in London.

I have the honor to serve alongside my peers in the Global CEO Initiative on AD. My passion as a scientist to find a therapy to mitigate the medical effects of this terrible disease is matched by my determination to engage with key policymakes such as yourselves to pull together all the key elements of a Global Action Plan similar to that the world established 30 years ago when faced with the HIV/AIDS epidemic. In my view, the challenges of AD today are on the same scale, if not greater.

Let me start the session with some hard basic facts on AD:

- AD is an irreversible degeneration of the brain that causes a loss of memory, cognition, personality and other functions that eventually lead to death.
- AD is not a normal part of aging but its occurrence correlates with aging
- There is no cure.
- According to the World Health Organization and Alzheimer's Disease International 2012 Dementia Report, it is estimated that there were 35.6 million people with dementia, including Alzheimer's disease, worldwide in 2010. This number is projected to nearly double every 20 years, increasing to 65.7 million in 2030 and 115.4 million in 2050.[1]
- With an ageing population, the prevalence of AD is estimated to continue to grow across Europe at about the same pace as in the US.
- Several countries, including France, Australia and England, have specific plans in place to address dementia, including Alzheimer's disease.[1]

RESEARCH AND DEVELOPMENT CHALLENGES:

As a researcher and a CEO, my specific role today is to share with you some challenges of the research and development in Alzheimer's disease. Even more than a century after it was first observed, today we still do not know the exact causes of the disease and the exact molecular basis. We do know that AD is characterized by the loss of neurons and synapses which translates into loss of brain volume and atrophy of certain regions of the brain. We also know that two proteins – Beta-amyloid and Tau – are shown to be ultimately involved in the disease process.
The goal of the research is to find a total cure. Alzheimer's disease (AD) might be treated with symptomatic, neuroprotective, or neurorestorative therapies. Neuroprotective and neurorestorative interventions are disease-modifying therapies, none of which exist today. Disease modification can be defined as treatments or interventions that affect the underlying pathophysiology of the disease and have a beneficial outcome on the course of AD. In a clinical trial the criteria for affecting the underlying cause of the disease can be supported by demonstrating an effect on a biomarker such as medial temporal atrophy on magnetic resonance imaging (MRI) or diminished tau or phospho-tau levels in cerebrospinal fluid. A delay in onset of 5 years starting 2015 results in US$ 447 billion saving of total expected costs of US$ 1.078 billion in the US alone.

One of the stumbling blocks of AD treatment is the time of intervention. Learning from the failures of recent drugs in clinical development, there is scientific consensus that early presymptomatic intervention appears to be the best shot. As you would imagine, delivering a therapy to people before they are even showing signs of the illness or when the illness may be in its earliest forms poses another significant challenge in designing and implementing clinical trials and in recruiting patients.

---

[1] Alzheimer's Disease International, World Health Organization. Dementia: A Public Health Priority. April 2012. http://www.who.int/mental_health/publications/dementia_report_2012.

This makes early and accurate diagnosis and clinical trial recruitment infrastructure imperative to our efforts at achieving success.

Today, clinical testing assessing (memory function) is still the state-of-the-art methodology; there has been a great effort to ease and standardized these clinical protocols for practicing physicians. The only definite diagnosis is post–mortem when brain material is available and the tangles can be histological examined (Braak stages).Recently important advances have been made in Neuroimaging which provides prognostic value for disease diagnosis and progression. However, Neuroimaging is very expensive and not yet easily accessible.

Biomarkers have the potential to help better identify Alzheimer's patients during the pre-symptomatic stages of the disease. They have proven to be vital in therapy development efforts, particularly when dealing with a disease as complex as Alzheimer's because they help researchers understand whether or not a potential therapy is having an impact sure of an outright cure or reversal of a disease. A commonly understood biomarker would be cholesterol levels. We know that high cholesterol is a driver of heart disease. Therefore, we know that medications, like statins that lower cholesterol levels, can be effective in reducing one's risk for heart disease. Another example would be the viral load or the level of HIV in a person's blood. Medications today exist to lower a person's viral load and, in so doing, control the virus. While biomarkers are quite helpful, qualifying or validating a biomarker so that it is widely accepted by the research community and by regulators – such as at the EMA and the FDA who will be reviewing a drug to determine if it is safe and effective – is a challenge in the Alzheimer's space, a challenge that must be tackled.

Really important advances have been made in neuroimaging and biomarker research. However, their validation for disease diagnosis and progress as well as their utility of assessment of drug responses is still ongoing.

On 31 October, the European Medicines Agency (EMA) released a concept paper on the need to revise the guideline on medicines for the treatment of Alzheimer's disease and other dementias for public consultation.

New research diagnostic criteria are being used in clinical trials for different stages of the disease. In addition, a number of biomarkers to help identify and select patients at the pre-dementia stage of the disease have been developed by medicines developers; several have received a qualification opinion from the Agency's Committee for Medicinal Products for Human Use (CHMP) for use in the development of medicines.

The concept paper describes how these new developments have had an impact on recent and future clinical-trial protocols and discusses the elements to consider as part of the revision of the current guideline. These include the:

- Impact of new diagnostic criteria for Alzheimer's disease, including early and even asymptomatic disease stages on clinical-trial design;
- Choice of parameters to measure trial outcomes and the need for distinct assessment tools for the different disease stages in Alzheimer's (different signs and symptoms, differences in change over time, severity);
- Assessment of efficacy and safety in different age groups;
- Potential use of biomarkers and their temporal relationship with the different phases of Alzheimer's disease at different stages of medicine development (mechanism of action, use as diagnostic test, enrichment of study populations, stratification of subgroups, safety and efficacy markers, etc.);
- Design of long-term efficacy and safety studies;
  Usefulness of combination therapy and corresponding study designs.

THE G8 DEMENTIA SUMMIT AND BEYOND:

In Europe AD has been put on the priority agenda of many governments. The health ministers from the G8 nations will meet the first ever global summit on dementia to help improve management of the disease and accelerate the development of new treatments under the leadership of the UK government.
Prime Minister David Cameron and Health Secretary Jeremy Hunt said they will use the UK's presidency of the G8 this year to spearhead "coordinated global action" against one of the greatest current healthcare challenges. I applaud Prime Minister Cameron for this leadership and urge other G8 nations to support this work at the highest level possible.

The high-level summit, which is to be held in London on December 11, will host discussion to shape an effective international solution to dementia, including looking for effective therapies and responses to slow dementia's impact.

The G8 have a unique chance to help people manage dementia better, lead healthier lives and deliver real improvements in care and substantial economic savings.

Currently, someone is diagnosed with dementia every four seconds around the globe and the disease costs more than $650 billion a year. While 70% of this cost is incurred in 'medically advanced' nations like Western Europe and North America, nearly 60% of people with the condition live in developing countries.

The four pillars of the G8 Dementia Summit are the followings:

1. **Building cooperation networks among governments, regulators, the private sector and the nonprofits.**
2. **Coordination in business leading to prevention of dementia.**
3. **Investment in solutions and treatments.**
4. **Laying the foundations for a transition to an aging society without dementia.**

I am particularly enthusiastic and optimistic about the potential for greater levels of public-private partnership not limited to one nation or region but rather spanning the world. Such efforts are necessary if we are to achieve our shared goals of defeating Alzheimer's disease. Alzheimer's and dementia affect the entire globe and do not recognize national borders. It is a global crisis that merits a global response.

Beyond the CEO Initiative and the G8 Summit, let me provide you with a brief update on some other encouraging developments happening primarily here in Europe.

European Commission

European Innovation Partnership on Active and Healthy Ageing (EIP) is a new stakeholder-driven approach to innovation, whose overarching target is to add two years to the average number of healthy life years in the European Union by the year 2020.

The Partnership is in its implementation phase: more than 3,000 partners are involved in mobilizing efforts and resources to carry forward the EIP 6 action plans:

- Prescription and adherence to treatment
- Personalized health management: Falls prevention
- Prevention of functional decline and frailty
- Integrated care for chronic diseases, including remote monitoring at regional level
- Interoperable independent living solutions
- Age friendly buildings, cities and environments

Private Public Partnership for AD Clinical Trials (EPOC-AD)

Greater cooperation and collaboration between academia, government and industry could enhance the drug development process. A public-private partnership is proposed to promote more efficient clinical trial designs and execution of clinical trials aimed at preventing AD dementia. The plan would create a precompetitive space to enable collaboration for optimizing patient selection, clinical trials methodologies, and candidate therapies, as well as conducting adaptive clinical trials that will produce the greatest likelihood of success.

The mission of EPOC-AD is therefore to advance this novel collaborative partnership and drive a more successful approach to drug development for preventing AD dementia. The goal is to enable rapid cycling of learning from registries and longitudinal cohorts into adaptive clinical trials that shorten timelines, improve efficiencies and permit more rapid dissemination of knowledge. A consortium of industrial, governmental and academic partners will be formed to advance this research program

EPOC-AD will conduct a continuous, global, multicenter and multi-agent clinical trial designed to efficiently identify treatments, or combinations of treatments, with sufficient promise for the prevention of halting of progression of AD to warrant definitive confirmatory testing. Basically, the trial will serve as an efficient and rigorous screen or gateway prior to confirmatory standalone trials.

CONCLUSION:

In conclusion, it is my earnest desire to convey to the Committee that we need the inspiring leadership of the United States government to play a key role and be a role model in facing one of the most severe and complex challenges of the 21st century. The US could play a cohesive role in helping to join hands through the G8 Summit, extending the message across to the OECD. The CEOi can be the key catalyst of all of these efforts.

Thank you again for this hearing. Although many differences exist within the international community, we share an important goal: finding a cure for Alzheimer's disease and eliminating the personal, financial and social burdens of this terrible disease. I remain confident that with united forces and the lead of your nation in a Global Action Plan, we can achieve this goal.

Mr. SMITH. Dr. Pfeifer, thank you very much for taking the time to address our subcommittee and by extension the U.S. Congress, and thank you for your extraordinary work on behalf of Alzheimer's patients.

A couple of questions that I would like to just raise. Do any of our panelists have a sense as to where—everyone asks me in my district and I get this every time I am out on the road particularly when I am speaking about Alzheimer's. How close are we to a breakthrough on delaying early onset, certainly recognizing it, but the drugs that are in the mix that are in the pipeline, is there reason for serious hope that we may be many years away or maybe just a few? What is your sense on that?

Mr. VRADENBURG. I will give you a view, but I would be very interested in both the Association and Andrea's view since this is obviously unscripted. There are several drugs in late stages of development in the pipeline. They are targeted at mild to moderate cases of dementia and have not yet been targeted to earlier cases, at least in the current late-stage trials. And they are showing a modicum of possibility that we could slow down the rate of decline. Those drugs are going to be finishing trials in the roughly 2015–2016 time frame. They will be before, if those trials are successful, the FDA in the 2016–1017 time frame, and it is possible that we will have a first generation drug for mild to moderate victims of this disease in that time frame.

The world as Dr. Pfeifer has laid out has now begun to shift its attention to earlier stages of the disease, so the same drug that is now in trials for mild to moderate dementia is now going into trial for much earlier stages of dementia, and if those prove successful then we will have a drug on the market that may be potentially administerable to patients before they get any signs of cognitive or functional decline, and on the current timeline that would probably be in 2018 to 2020 time frame. But I have always said to treat it as the metaphor of what happens when you try and introduce a new product. The first time you get a new product it is clunky, it is expensive. The second generation of that product is better, it will be less expensive, it will be more effective.

So while I think there is reason for confidence that by 2020 we will have a drug on the market that will have a modest effect on the progression of this disease, I think that the prospect of getting a truly effective means of prevention and treatment is possible, perhaps even likely by 2025, but quite frankly, dependents highly on funding and focus between now and then. So I think this is not something that by 2025 is going to happen with business as usual. It is going to require increased focus and increased resource in order to get us there.

Mr. SMITH. Thank you.

Mr. BAUMGART. I would say I am cautiously optimistic, but I would underscore what George said at the end of his statement. I think that the scientific community has the ideas, the will is there, the technology is there. What is lacking is the level of resources and the commitment that is necessary to get us there. And so I am optimistic that we can, but it will require a greater commitment.

The National Plan, as you know, includes a goal of effectively treating and preventing Alzheimer's by 2025. There will be interim steps. There will be interim progress. And one of the great developments of the National Plan so far is that the National Institutes of Health finally has a blueprint; it has timelines; and it has milestones for us to reach that goal. So I think the question now is whether we will, and the government will, come through with the resources that are necessary.

Mr. SMITH. Dr. Pfeifer, did you want to speak to that?

Ms. PFEIFER. Yes. I just would like to add maybe one aspect which I consider is enormously important for the progress we need. As it was mentioned by George and previously also by myself, the world is changing from intervention treatment trials to prevention trials because obviously the biggest impact on society would be if we could actually prevent the disease rather than treat the disease. Now as we all know there is no diagnostic means today available which would allow us to actually select the patients which would eventually get the disease. So the only way to do that is actually to work with genetically predisposed population, like, for example, the Colombia population, in order to really test if prevention is possible.

So my wish, my dream, would be to have concerted actions and funding to support research toward biomarkers and better diagnostic means. Because only if we can, in fact, enhance the early diagnostics, so diagnostic before the disease started, only then we can really think about prevention trial which would really change result. So we need more funding for doing research in this important area.

Mr. SMITH. Yes?

Mr. BAUMGART. I would just add, Mr. Chairman, that the greatest obstacle to progress after funding is the number of people who are not participating in clinical trials. We need a lot more participants in clinical trials, not only those with the disease, but when it comes to things like prevention trials, we need healthy individuals to enroll in clinical trials as well. And I know there are some efforts underway, and the Alzheimer's Association has a trial match program to try to encourage this. But efforts by the government to encourage greater participation in clinical trials are also important if we are going to get there.

Mr. SMITH. As I think we all know, the U.N. estimates for growth in population is almost always about aging. When we climb to 9 billion or thereabouts, maybe even 10 billion, it is not about children it is about aging, and people are living longer, which is all the more reason why the call and the action plans have to be put into place now as never before, which is why we are having this hearing.

I wanted to ask you a couple of very quick questions. We have an hour's worth of voting on the floor that just started and so I will ask a few questions and then yield to Mr. Weber because I don't want to have you sit here and wait a full hour. But the amount of money, the billion dollars that you mentioned earlier, Mr. Vradenburg. We have tried, as you know, for years, and we worked very closely with both of you, frankly, to try to get the Alzheimer's Breakthrough Act passed, to get it up to at least $750 billion of NIH funding, and we fall far short all the time despite herculean efforts, bipartisan to the core.

How many good—and Dr. Pfeifer you might speak to this as well from the European side—how many laudable proposals fall off the table at NIH or any other research facility or funding mechanism because the money isn't there? I remember hearing that one estimate was like three out of four. So we are missing the opportunity to find what may be as close to a brass ring as it could be because that project and that focus and that research proposal did not get funded. If you could speak to that.

Mr. VRADENBURG. Well, I think the number is a lot greater than that. The current payline is in the teens, which means one out of six or one out of seven is getting approved, and those are of projects that have gone through peer review and been successful. And the only reason that it is even that high is that the NIH has cut back the amount of those grants so that the numbers, if you took the level of grants that were funded several years ago, the number of approved grants would be under 10 percent. So we are talking about a situation where one in six or seven, perhaps one in ten depending on the size of the grant, has currently been approved. And those are peer reviewed grants that are found to have been meritorious.

Your point, Mr. Chairman, one additional point. This is beyond a health issue as just pointed out by the Sec on Aging. At our recent Alzheimer's Disease Summit: The Path to 2025 that we conducted in New York, a member of the Japanese cabinet came to speak. And her country is beginning to shift its entire economic strategy from one of manufacturing to one of service because they are not going to have enough workers at working age populations in order to support their manufacturing economy. So over a period of years, they are having to shift their entire national economic strategy to less labor intensive jobs, jobs that can be performed by older individuals and potentially even older individuals from their homes.

So this is an issue of health as Matthew has pointed out dramatically, but it is an economic imperative for countries as their age shifts. Western Europe is going through this in spades on how to adjust to this. And of course, the entitlement cost spending going through the roof, in part because of this, suggests that this is a fiscal issue as well. So it is a health issue. We have not been able yet to engage economic ministers and finance ministers in understanding the import of an aging world on the shifts in relative economic strengths of different countries.

We have seen China change its policy on the one-child policy because it foresees itself running out of workers in 20 to 30 years. So they are beginning to adjust their social policies to respond to the demographic changes that you just referred to. So this is a very, very significant thing for the relative economic power of countries around the world in the coming two to three to four decades.

Mr. SMITH. Mr. Weber?

Mr. WEBER. Thank you, Mr. Chairman. This question is for the panel. Other countries that are involved, engaged alongside of the United States, if you will, in this fight? Top three?

Mr. BAUMGART. I would say France was one of the first countries to develop a national plan, and when Mr. Sarkozy was President there was a commitment from the topmost levels of government to actually carry out the plan. I would also say the United Kingdom has a fairly robust and increasing research program and a commitment to funding research. So those would be my top two.

Mr. WEBER. There is not a third one?

Mr. VRADENBURG. I would add Canada. Although it is not a significant size, they are very actively, very well organized.

Mr. WEBER. Okay. Yes, ma'am.

Ms. PFEIFER. Yes. Thank you, Mr. Chairman. Sweden also has an extremely well-defined plan for Alzheimer's. One of her, I would say, leading ones in Europe.

Mr. WEBER. Okay, thank you. You mentioned costs associated with Alzheimer's. Is there a per capita cost that has been demonstrated and nailed down and calculated? What does it cost per capita in the United States? What does it cost per capita in Switzerland? What does it cost per capita in France and UK?

Mr. BAUMGART. So I haven't actually calculated the per capita costs. You could calculate it. The estimates are that the total cost of caring for people with Alzheimer's and dementia in the United States this year will be $203 billion. So I haven't actually done the math, but you could do the math from that.

Mr. VRADENBURG. One of the things that the Alzheimer's Association did very well, they did a study a few years ago, Mr. Weber, in which they looked at the costs to Medicare of a patient with dementia, a beneficiary with dementia and one without dementia. And the cost to the Medicare system is three times greater for a beneficiary with Alzheimer's than a beneficiary without Alzheimer's. And with respect to Medicaid, it is 19.

Mr. BAUMGART. It is 19.

Mr. VRADENBURG. 19 times more expensive to Medicaid to have a beneficiary with Alzheimer's than a beneficiary without Alzheimer's.

Mr. WEBER. And Dr. Pfeifer, in Switzerland, same question.

Ms. PFEIFER. Yes. So there are some numbers. The last numbers which I saw were 60,000 euros per person per year, so per patient per year. So it is a substantial amount of money.

Mr. WEBER. Can you translate the euros into dollars for me?

Mr. VRADENBURG. It is about $100,000.

Mr. WEBER. About $100,000. Okay. What would you say is the main focus of the preventive research? Are we looking at brain health, circulatory health, neurons? What is the main focus of that research?

Mr. BAUMGART. I think there are a lot of areas of focus. Operating on the principle that what is good for your heart is good for your brain, there is a lot of research on physical activity and whether that can slow the progression or even prevent the disease, if the physical activity is regular and vigorous in middle age. There are some studies on diet. In terms of brain health and physical health connection, there are smoking studies. There have been studies that show that smoking is also bad for your brain.

Mr. WEBER. As anybody with a brain should know that.

Mr. BAUMGART. Yes. And so you have a lot of focus on how do you make the connection between the physical and the mental. And one other area that is key is the connection between diabetes and Alzheimer's. We do know there is a connection. Scientists aren't quite sure exactly how the connection works, but we do know that you are at increased risk for Alzheimer's disease in later life if you have diabetes in mid-life. So that is another area of ongoing research.

Mr. VRADENBURG. So the primary focus has been around a protein called beta-amyloid, and I believe that there is a cascading effect that occurs with some misfolded proteins that begin to accumulate into beta-amyloid and then into tau and then through inflammation into the death of neurons and synapses. And one of the confounding things here is that there are many people who live very healthy and very cognitively active lives well into their 90s who have a lot of beta-amyloid in their brain, and indeed a lot with beta-amyloid and tau.

And so what scientists are now focusing on as the key trigger is an inflammatory response that builds off of that. So the science is looking not just at how to regulate better the beta-amyloid and tau buildup in the brain, but also potentially at what is maybe protective, in protecting those people with beta-amyloid and tau not turning into cognitive disabled people. So they are looking both at the mechanisms of stopping the bad stuff and promoting the good stuff.

Mr. WEBER. And Dr. Pfeifer, would you like to weigh in?

Ms. PFEIFER. No, I think George perfectly explained what is, I would say, most advanced belief in what would be the best targets to cure, hold or prevent the disease. I think what becomes quite obvious is the basic interaction between the beta-amyloid and tau. So maybe we actually have to really tackle both proteins together in combination therapies in order to really have the benefit of the momentary drug development. A third aspect comes in. There seems to be quite a few, in fact 30 percent of Alzheimer's patients have also some aspects of Parkinson's. There is another protein, which is alpha-synuclein, and this protein seems to be also involved. So I think when we are looking forward is really to focus on how are these different elements working together, and it seems more and more important that you think about combinational therapies not just monotherapies.

And maybe a last aspect, of course I am referring to my past. I was actually doing the first Alzheimer's study with food, medical food, and I do believe that the aspect of utilizing beneficial foods could be strengthened, because I am absolutely convinced that prevention could also come from the food area. And this is maybe an area which we have a bit neglected in the past.

Mr. WEBER. Okay, thank you. That is it, Mr. Chairman, I am going to head for vote.

Mr. SMITH. We are actually out of time. And I apologize, but I do have just one final comment, two comments I want to make.

One, Mr. Vradenburg, your thought of more parliamentarians connecting, I think, is a great one. I am the co-chairman of the Helsinki Commission, the Commission on Security and Cooperation in Europe, and we have resolutions and meetings three times a year. The big one is July. As a result, I think your recommendation is a good one, I plan on, I will offer a resolution to try to get each of the parliamentarians, and usually about 300 show up from 57 countries so it is not insignificant, to take back this urgent call, and by then we will have the G–8 summit, hopefully a very strong plan of action in a cascading way to keep building out this need.

I went back and looked at a bill that I had introduced working very closely with the Alzheimer's Association and with you, George, as well, called the Ronald Reagan Alzheimer's Breakthrough Act of 2005. And the number that we had in there for NIH was $1.4 billion. And unfortunately, in real dollars we have actually gone down from where it was then. So it is maybe not exactly, but in no way has it approximated the need that exists in marrying up the resources to make sure.

And your point, Mr. Vradenburg, about one out of six, it may be even worse, peer reviewed proposals dropping off the table and not getting funded, that is unconscionable, frankly. So we need to do more. We hope to do more. As you know, Maxine Waters and I, we are co-chairs of the caucus. Ed Markey who was the co-chair for years is now over on the Senate side doing his good work there.

So this hearing launches into G–8, launches into what do we do as a Congress, and hopefully like combating HIV/AIDS pandemic, we will come out of the blocks as never before to tackle and combat and hopefully eradicate this horrible disease, or at least make serious strides in early onset and dealing with the issue. So thank you so very much. Do you have any final comments?

Mr. VRADENBURG. Thank you. Thank you, Chairman Smith, for your leadership in this space and I look forward to working with you both domestically and internationally on this issue.

Mr. BAUMGART. Thank you, Mr. Chairman.

Mr. SMITH. Thank you so much. Dr. Pfeifer, thank you so much——

Ms. PFEIFER. Thank you.

Mr. SMITH [continuing]. For coming in from the continent of Europe.

Let me just finally also say before I, we will take everything you have said, your testimonies are outstanding. We will get them to Secretary Sebelius and all the others at HHS with a letter signed in a bipartisan way with my ranking member, and ask them to really seriously look—I know you have other avenues to get through to them, but let them know that we are watching as well and we are advocates, as are you. But thank you so much. The hearing is adjourned.

[Whereupon, at 11:12 a.m., the subcommittee was adjourned.]

APPENDIX

MATERIAL SUBMITTED FOR THE RECORD

SUBCOMMITTEE HEARING NOTICE
COMMITTEE ON FOREIGN AFFAIRS
U.S. HOUSE OF REPRESENTATIVES
WASHINGTON, DC 20515-6128

Subcommittee on Africa, Global Health, Global Human Rights, and International Organizations
Christopher H. Smith (R-NJ), Chairman

November 20, 2013

TO: MEMBERS OF THE COMMITTEE ON FOREIGN AFFAIRS

You are respectfully requested to attend an OPEN hearing of the Committee on Foreign Affairs, to be held by the Subcommittee on Africa, Global Health, Global Human Rights, and International Organizations in Room 2172 of the Rayburn House Office Building (and available live on the Committee website at www.foreignaffairs.house.gov):

DATE: Thursday, November 21, 2013

TIME: 10:15 a.m.

SUBJECT: The Global Challenge of Alzheimer's: The G-8 Dementia Summit and Beyond

WITNESSES: Andrea Pfeifer, Ph.D.
Chief Executive Officer
AC Immune
(Appearing via videoconference)

Mr. George Vradenburg
Chairman and Founder
USAgainstAlzheimer's

Mr. Matthew Baumgart
Senior Director of Public Policy
Alzheimer's Association

By Direction of the Chairman

COMMITTEE ON FOREIGN AFFAIRS

MINUTES OF SUBCOMMITTEE ON _Africa, Global Health, Global Human Rights, and International Organizations_ HEARING

Day___ _Thursday_____ Date__ _November 21, 2013___ Room _2172 Rayburn HOB_

Starting Time __ _10:15 a.m._ Ending Time ___ _11:11 a.m._

Recesses | _0_ | (____to____) (____to____) (____to____) (____to____) (____to____) (____to____)

Presiding Member(s)

Rep. Chris Smith

Check all of the following that apply:

Open Session ☑
Executive (closed) Session ☐
Televised ☑

Electronically Recorded (taped) ☑
Stenographic Record ☑

TITLE OF HEARING:

The Global Challenge of Alzheimer's: The G-8 Dementia Summit and Beyond

SUBCOMMITTEE MEMBERS PRESENT:

Rep. Randy Weber, Rep. Ami Bera

NON-SUBCOMMITTEE MEMBERS PRESENT: _(Mark with an * if they are not members of full committee.)_

HEARING WITNESSES: Same as meeting notice attached? Yes ☑ No ☐
(If "no", please list below and include title, agency, department, or organization.)

STATEMENTS FOR THE RECORD: _(List any statements submitted for the record.)_

Prepared statement from Rep. Maxine Waters

TIME SCHEDULED TO RECONVENE _____
or
TIME ADJOURNED ___ _11:11 a.m._

Gregory D. Simpkins
Subcommittee Staff Director

"The Global Challenge of Alzheimer's: The G-8 Dementia Summit and Beyond"

House Committee on Foreign Affairs

Subcommittee on Africa, Global Health, Global Human Rights, and International Organizations

Statement by Rep. Maxine Waters

November 21, 2013

I would like to thank Chairman Chris Smith, my Republican Co-Chair of the Congressional Task Force on Alzheimer's Disease, as well as Ranking Member Karen Bass, for organizing this hearing and inviting me to participate.

This hearing, "The Global Challenge of Alzheimer's: The G-8 Dementia Summit and Beyond," addresses an important topic. As the Democratic Co-Chair of the Congressional Task Force on Alzheimer's Disease, I know how devastating Alzheimer's and other forms of dementia can be for individuals and families.

Alzheimer's and other forms of dementia primarily affect the elderly. As populations age, more individuals are likely to be affected by these conditions. According to the World Health Organization, Alzheimer's disease is the most common form of dementia, accounting for 60 to 70 percent of dementia cases worldwide.

Here in the United States, Alzheimer's disease is the sixth leading cause of death, and it affects over five million American families. One in nine Americans age 65 and older has Alzheimer's, and one in three Americans age 85 and older suffers from this disease. The Alzheimer's Association estimates that more than 7 million Americans over age 65 will have Alzheimer's by the year 2025. Every 68 seconds, another person in the United States develops Alzheimer's.

Most Americans suffering from Alzheimer's disease live at home under the care of family and friends. More than 15 million Americans provide unpaid care for a person with Alzheimer's disease or another form of dementia. Caregivers include spouses, children, and grandchildren. Caregivers face a variety of challenges, ranging from assisting patients with feeding, bathing, and dressing to helping them take their medications, managing their finances, and making legal decisions.

Alzheimer's and other forms of dementia present growing challenges not just in the United States but also in many countries around the world. According to data compiled by the Congressional Research Service, more than 35 million people worldwide suffered from dementia in 2010. By the year 2050, that number is expected to increase by 224 percent to more than 115 million people.

The first G-8 Dementia Summit will be held on December 11th in the United Kingdom. The purpose of the summit is to bring health ministers, researchers, physicians, industry leaders, and others together to discuss how they can coordinate efforts and shape an effective international solution to dementia.

The World Health Organization estimates that more than half of global dementia cases are in low- and middle-income countries. The Congressional Research Service projected that by 2050, there will be 8.7 million people with dementia in Africa, 16.1 million people with dementia in Latin America, 29.2 million people with dementia in South/Southeast Asia, and 30.8 million people with dementia in East Asia.

Alzheimer's disease and other dementias present special challenges in low- and middle-income countries. In high-income countries, institutions like nursing homes provide care for many of the individuals who are suffering from dementia, and programs like Medicare, Medicaid, and social services for seniors provide financial support to families struggling to care for an affected loved one. However, in most low- and middle-income countries, public medical and social services for people with dementia are rare. Consequently, care for individuals with dementia in these countries is predominantly the responsibility of their families.

Countries that have been heavily impacted by HIV/AIDS face additional challenges in dealing with dementia. Millions of children have been orphaned by HIV/AIDS, and grandparents play an important role in raising many of these children. According to UNAIDS, nearly 17 million children worldwide have lost at least one parent to HIV/AIDS, and almost 90 percent of them live in Africa. UNAIDS further estimates that, in some countries, more than half of all children who lost a parent to HIV/AIDS are being cared for by a grandparent. The difficulties for families and communities could be tremendous if some of these grandparents who are caring for their grandchildren begin to develop dementia and need care themselves.

These are just a few of the many challenges that increasing rates of Alzheimer's and dementia could pose to the international community. I hope that the G-8 Dementia Summit will give the international community an opportunity to discuss these challenges and begin to develop comprehensive strategies to address them. I support the participation of U.S. officials in the Summit, and I look forward to hearing their report on the Summit's achievements.

Once again, I thank my colleagues, Chairman Smith and Ranking Member Bass, for allowing me to participate in this hearing, and I look forward to discussing the G-8 Dementia Summit with them and working to alleviate the global burden of Alzheimer's disease and dementia.

www.ingramcontent.com/pod-product-compliance
Lightning Source LLC
Chambersburg PA
CBHW052019280526
45793CB00005B/1037